Who Hit the Down Button?

Life with a Chronic Illness or Disability

by

Phyllis Porter Dolislager

Copyright © 2023, 2018, 2009, 2008
By Phyllis Porter Dolislager

Who Hit the Down Button
Life with a Chronic Illness or Disability

Printed in the United States

All rights reserved. No part of this publication may be reproduced or transmitted in any form or by any means without written permission of the author.

ISBN-13: 978-1721085729

ISBN-10: 1721085726

To purchase additional copies of this book and other books by the author, visit Amazon.com.

While reading this short book I found myself wishing that this woman was a next-door neighbor, an easily accessible friend to talk with and influence my life with her gentility and acceptance. I had polio too, and much of what she has written here about her life after polio parallels my own, especially her feelings of insecurity and aloneness. Phyllis has lived her life with grace; I've lived my life fighting the damn effects of the disease. Her attitude has been better, and I encourage you to read this book to find out why.

Robert Arnold
Polio Survivor

Phyllis Dolislager writes from a heart filled with a lifetime of struggling with a progressive physical condition. In the face of such a challenge, she raised a family, served on the mission field, and has written volumes that speak to the heart of other struggling people. Feeling uplifted is not an option for readers of this work; it will be automatic.

Dr. David R. Miller
Psychologist

This book is an act of love. As a life-long dedicated communicator and teacher, Phyllis Dolislager shares her experiences of Post-Polio, along with those of her supporters, with heart-warming—sometimes heart wrenching—anecdotes and lessons that instill hope and encourage conscious choice in patients and caregivers alike. Incorporating discussion questions and meditation topics for everyone with a chronic illness or physical disability, Phyllis's spirit and vitality shine through her writing. She inspires as she writes. She is a life example to us all.

Gail Powell, PhD
Massage Therapist, Chronic Illness

Author and former college professor, Phyllis Dolislager is no stranger to the unexpected challenges faced by those who live with an on-going physical disability. As a polio survivor, Phyllis balanced her life as a wife, mother and working professional with a permanent physical limitation. In more recent years, the stress of this "balancing act" pushed her to a crisis point of exhaustion. Honest and homespun, this true account of a soul-searching transition offers something for anyone facing the panic of physical decline.

Tom Vander Molen, Paraplegic
Veteran Radio Broadcaster

Dedication

To all care-givers and spouses, who help us through each and every day.

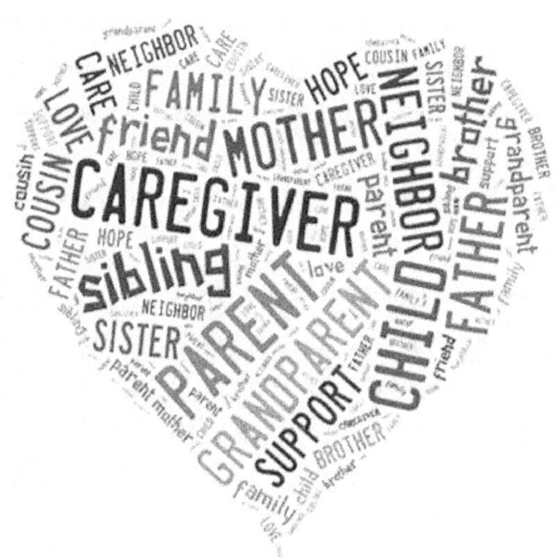

Preface

It had been my intent to write this book for some time, but life always seemed to get in the way. Since we first moved to Tennessee, I had written seven topics followed by three thought questions, but that was it. I never seemed to get any further.

However, when I started cleaning out the file cabinet I discovered that I had enough material already written to make this book. So, I put the articles in an order that seemed right to me. Then the idea came that I could add three questions after each one. And here you have it.

If you're reading this book by yourself, I hope you take the time to answer the questions in your own mind. If you're reading the book and then discussing it with others, use the questions as conversation starters. Let me know if there are other topics that you'd like added in a future edition.

As always, I couldn't do this without the help of my husband, Ron. He's the one who gets me through my daily life and even encourages my creative life. I love you, Ron.

This second edition has a change-out of polio survivor stories. Bruce and Diane and Maureen are friends that I met at the Boca Raton Post-Polio support group.

Encouraging Quotes

*I refused to lie down. I have my dark days, but
I don't ask, "Why me?" I ask, "What now?"*
--Daryl Mitchell

What doesn't destroy me makes me stronger –
Dr. Martin Luther King, Jr.

Your right hand upholds me.
--Psalm 18:35

*The only real invalid is the person who thinks she
or he is one.*
--Margaret Blackstone

*Most people are either busy dying ... or busy
living.*
--Joni Eareckson Tada

Contents

Who Pushed the "Down" Button?
Feelings about a chronic illness

I always knew that I was living on an elevator.
I remember stopping at certain floors.
Some I anticipated like teaching and giving
my Writing Workshops.
I wanted to stay and browse there all day.
A couple of times I'd inadvertently, I think, gotten off
at the wrong floor.
What in the world was I doing participating in a mock jury?
Testing mouthwashes?
Handing out food samples?
Oh, yes; now I remember.
I was between jobs, and any extra money was appreciated.

Some of the floors held more for me than others, and I
always did enjoy finding specials.
The linens and dishes fascinated me. I loved them all.
And then there was the shoe floor. I visited there often. Having a
size-7 right foot, and a size-10 left foot, shoe shopping became a
challenge, until … I found Jean, in Minnesota (now Arizona),
who had the exact opposite size feet as mine.

As the elevator continued to climb ever upward, reaching new
floors,
I added another degree behind my name.

We had lived … in Africa … for two years!
Then we moved to Florida.

And all too soon we were traveling again …
to our sons' weddings … then to their children's baptisms.
But … somewhere … in the busyness … I
lost track of which floor I was on … and what
I was looking for ….

In fact, I woke up one day, and the elevator, my trusty source of
motivation and transport was ….
Going … down!

What happened?
Who changed directions on me?
I'm not used to this downward motion.
I DON'T LIKE IT.
Oh God, did I do something wrong?
What is this?
I'm not working … or … shopping … or even
sleeping very well.
Where's my social life? I miss it. And what
is this pain all about?
When did this all happen?
How did I change directions without even knowing it?

The change was gradual, for a while.
The tension sneaked up and climbed onto my shoulders.
I woke up with chest pains.
I brought my work home and thought about it 24/7.
Even on vacation ….
I will never forget sitting in the Sheraton Hotel, overlooking
Niagara Falls, reading a Federal RFP—request for proposal.
(I was directing a teen pregnancy and STD prevention
program and always looking for funds.)

OK, so I did stop and stay too long on some floors,
but I don't remember the elevator changing directions. I
just remember the fatigue, lying on the couch after work,
and wishing for a massage every day.

I now know that I changed directions about 2001.
I also know that I can't do today what I could do a year ago …
or even six months ago.
Has the speed of the down elevator accelerated?
More than once the thought crossed my mind that I
wished I had a wheelchair because walking had
become such an effort.
I also know that my dream of going to Paris won't happen—
unless it's in a wheelchair.

Ron does the grocery shopping, or I
have them delivered. I can shop for
10 items or less,
but the last time I shopped for a week's worth of groceries, I had
fatigue and muscle weakness for two days.
And just last week,
I had to have someone start cleaning house for me. If
I need clothes, I can go to only one store, and I hope
and pray that they'll have what I need, in my size, at
my price.
I never thought that my shopping genes would be affected.

Polio.
Yes, it's affected my life since I was 18 months old. I've
spent 70 years working around it … overcoming it …
trying to forget it.

BUT it's become a guest who's outstayed its welcome. It's hard
to know what to do with it …
and its consequences.

Now we use a new name: Post-Polio Syndrome,   or
the Late Effects of Polio. 1.3 million of us in the
U.S. have it.
One friend calls it, "The gift that keeps on giving."

Like it or not, we have no choice but to accept its "gifts" of knee
braces, canes, pain medications, wheelchairs or scooters, and our
loss of freedom and social activities.

*There are days that I literally grieve for my
former life on the "up" elevator.*

The prognosis, you ask?
There's little chance for improvement; the odds
are heavily weighted in the direction of a
downward spiral.
BUT my mind continues to spin out of control with ideas that my
body can no longer accomplish. This might be my biggest
frustration. YET if my mind were to lose its creativity,
I'd be devastated.
So, in the long run, I do have a lot to be thankful for.

Then there's my faith.
If I didn't firmly believe that God is the Blessed Controller of all
things,
I would be devastated.

In his book, *The Purpose Driven Life*, Rick Warren says,
"Your circumstances are temporary,
but your character will last forever."

Personally, I think that using "wheelchair" in the same sentence with my own name is building as much character as I could ever wish for. Believing that good can come out of bad, I'm waiting . . . not anticipating . . . but waiting . . . to see how this "character thing" plays out.

* * *

Even though my physical body is weak, My heart
for God is strong!

Entry in my Journal

* * *

1. When was it official that you had a chronic illness or disability?
2. What was your first reaction?
3. How long did it take for you to come to acceptance?
Have you come to acceptance?

Who's in Control?

My first experience in a wheelchair almost ended in divorce court. Knowing that I'd never make it on my polio feet for three days at the National Booksellers Convention, I gave in and got a manual wheelchair. My husband Ron, bless his heart, willingly agreed to be my pusher.

Immediately we found an obstacle just getting from our hotel to the Orlando Convention Center next door. Fortunately, I could get out of the chair as he carried it up/down five or six steps. We figured out where the elevators were in the Convention Center, despaired that there was so much carpeting, but how were we to know that the popular book *Men Are from Mars and Women Are from Venus* was going to be our main problem?

I had taken seven copies of my latest book proposal with me. Selling one's self and one's book idea in three to five sentences is a precise skill. Timing is key. Imagine having made a great presentation, followed by a positive response, handing over the proposal, saying good-bye, but not moving. And having this happen more than once . . ..

I knew right then and there that I needed my own power. This person had to regain some control over her life. Three days in a manual chair—even with the world's best husband standing behind me and pushing me—was all it took. Decision time was here. But what was the solution?

Then we attended the Abilities Expos in Ft. Lauderdale, Florida and Doug of T.D. Medical introduced us to the EZ Power Chair. I wanted one!

* * *

I circled the entire showroom of J.D. Medical without spotting the EZ Power Chair that I had ordered. All the personnel were busy at their desks, and my entrance hadn't caught the attention of even one of them. Ron was still parking the car, and I felt alone as I stood in this field of dark shadows. Everything looked black to me and contributed to my feeling of being a part of a dream … or was it a nightmare?

Suddenly, the enthusiasm I'd had about getting a power chair was gone. In fact, it now seemed like a hideous, bad idea. There was no way I wanted to associate myself with this blackness . . . this gloom … this ….

About the same time Ron came in the store, the owner Doug also appeared with a smile and asked if I'd seen my chair. Forcing some anticipation into my voice and onto my face, I honestly replied, "No." I didn't dare tell him that 60 seconds earlier I had changed my mind about owning and using a power chair. But sanity won out, and we loaded it into the trunk of the car and headed home.

* * *

At home I practiced by taking the chair down two blocks of sidewalk to the mailbox. My driving skills (prowess with the joy stick) were horrid. I kept running off the sidewalk onto the grass. Even our dog, which was accompanying Ron and me, worked to stay out of my way. My right arm was also hurting—badly. Ron switched the joystick to the left hand, and the trial by error down the sidewalk began anew that next evening. I wasn't much better;

for 62 years my left hand had never had to perform such precise movements.

Fortunately, I am still ambulatory for short distances and do not need to use the power chair that much in the house. But of course, I did give it a trial run. I learned a few things: carpeting and wheelchairs are not 100% compatible. And if I wanted to go into the kitchen, I needed to go around and through the living room and dining room, as the doorway from the hallway into the kitchen was a tight fit and not good for novice, lefthanded, joystick users. When and if I need to use the chair full time, we'll need to make some flooring changes and maybe widen a few doorways.

* * *

My first trip to the mall with my power chair will forever be burned into my memory. With my sore right arm (I now know that it's a torn rotator cuff.), there was no way I could lift the chair into and out of the car's trunk by myself. Even though the power chair breaks down into three pieces, the heaviest piece is 29 pounds. My dear friend Evie Opitz was visiting and offered to accompany me on my trip to the mall—my first in three years!!! This was going to be a BIG day.

First, we practiced taking the chair apart, putting it into the trunk, and then taking it out and assembling it again. With Ron and Evie's husband, Al, looking on and offering all kinds of verbal instruction, we hoped that we had it firmly in mind, and off to the mall we went.

We parked at the Sears end of the mall, opened the trunk, and together unloaded the parts of the chair, and assembled it. Then I sat in my chair, and we were off to do our shopping.

But alas, getting through the door into Sears wasn't all that easy. It felt like I had to literally go left, go right, go left, and go right until I wiggled my way into the store. It was with a sigh of relief that we finally began my long-awaited, shopping trip.

What looked like "forward march" immediately became a "mine field." As I passed by a round table with a long, blue skirt, it started shedding small boxes of jewelry. They tumbled off falling randomly about me. I stopped, but I couldn't see that I owned any responsibility. I started to move, more boxes tumbled. I stopped, the boxes stopped. I'd start, and they'd throw themselves to the ground again.

Needing some assurance that I wasn't at fault, I looked around for Evie. There she was, immediately behind me, bent over in laughter. I mean, she was holding her sides she was laughing so hard. Catching my eye, she said, "Stop. Turn it off." As I realized that I hadn't been able to even start shopping without causing destruction, I was ready to cry. But there was my usually dignified friend laughing her head off. And that calmed me down, and I was able to see the humor.

As she untangled the hem of the table skirt from my chair's axle, she continued to laugh. So instead of retreating to the car, I continued our "forward march" past numerous brightly colored tables with skirts holding more boxes of jewelry.

Three hours later, with our purchases stuffed into the storage area under my seat, we headed back through Sears to the car. This time we by-passed the skirted, "mine field," and I even made it through the doorway without bouncing back and forth, hitting its sides.

As we disassembled the wheelchair and placed its parts, plus our packages, into the car's trunk, it was with a true sense of accomplishment and a smile on my face that I, the proud owner of a power chair, headed home.

* * *

1.   What adjustments have you had to make in your life?
2.   Do you remember a time when you could finally laugh at yourself despite your problems? What was it?
3.   Who has helped you along the way?

We Are Survivors

Inspired by Jody Taylor who said,
I should have gotten this powered wheelchair two years ago.

Long before we'd heard of body types, personality
profiles, or right brain/left brain— we finished what we'd
begun and always did our best. Work ethic. We had it.
We were survivors.

As we grew and matured, no one needed to encourage us.
We gave ourselves more pressure than we could handle. We
were Type A: hard-driving, time-conscious, overachieving
perfectionists.

We personified self-esteem. We knew all about drive.
We were survivors.

And then Post-Polio syndrome reared its ugly head, and
we tasted our first loss of confidence since contracting
polio.

And it was a major loss: our health, our bodies.
We were letting ourselves down; we were failing. This was
a new experience for us. We didn't know how to handle it.
We were survivors.

Embrace an assistive device? Take a nap? Ask for help?
What ridiculous mirage was this!
We were the survivors—not the losers.

It's taken us time to accept our new limitations.
We'd rather die in battle … than give up.

But one by one our Type A personalities have shifted to the opposite side of our brains, and we decided that if we were going to have a life . . . we needed to embrace our naps, use our assistive devices, and once again become survivors.

Now we buy minivans to transport our electric scooters and wheelchairs. We take vacations on accommodating cruise lines. And reluctantly we admit how stubborn we'd been not to accept the help that had been available to us years earlier.

We're still Type A. Our minds haven't stopped working. But now we're educating our younger doctors about Post Polio and striving for enforcement of the ADA Thank God, we still have a job to do!
We ARE survivors.

Written October 3 and 4, 2003 [1] Americans with Disabilities Act
   * * *

1. How has your personality type helped or hindered you in facing your challenges?
2. How do you keep your doctors up to date about your health?
3. What assistive devices do you use?

Special People

I think there will be a special place in heaven for caregivers.

Have you loaded wheelchairs into cars or vans or cut up food and gently placed it into your mate's mouth, or emptied bladder bags or positioned sleep machines? There must be a special place for you.

Have you stood in line to buy take-out or stopped for groceries on your way home from work? There's a special place in our hearts for you.

Have you held the hand of your ill, loved one and reminded them of why you chose to marry him/her in the first place? And then added the reasons why you'd do it all over again? There's a special reward in heaven for you.

You may think that no one knows, and no one cares or understands, but you're wrong, my friend.

Remember, Scripture says, "Show mercy and compassion to one another."   Zechariah 7:9

This week hold your head a little higher and place a smile on your face. For someone sees your acts of kindness— He cares, and He remembers.

10/27/03~ After dinner with Post-Polio friends

* * *

1. Do you have someone or an organization that helps you?
2. Describe an instance when you felt supported and nurtured in a time of need.
3. How did you express your appreciation?

Doctor's Appointments and Relationships

I make it a point to learn the nurses' names. (At this point, I write their names down by the doctors' phone numbers, as I can't remember them all.) I try to give them a cheery greeting and a positive comment on either their phone manners or how they treat me in person. They put up with so much negativity that my positive comment stands out.

This morning I went to get my flu shot at my G.P.'s. office. I stopped and bought a dozen bagels, two tubs of cream cheese, and a funny, thank you card for them. They loved it, and they treat me like they love me too.

When I offer them my books to read, they're always eager to take them because I've built a warm relationship with them. Somehow God has turned this sometimes negative or dreaded experience into a way for me to share my faith.

In my G.I. doctor's office, I once prayed with a nurse. Another time I witnessed such crazy going-on's in the waiting room, that I wrote a silly poem about it. It gave them all a good laugh, and once again they were willing to listen to me share snippets of my faith, and to accept my books. I've taken them bagels too, but they prefer my chocolate brownies.

And when it comes to getting free samples of meds, they give me a lot.

Also, one of the nurses, who I met when I had a colonoscopy, contacted me later to edit a manuscript for her.
It has turned out to be an on-going relationship and a good friendship.

I can't get out like I used to, so I find I need to build relationships whenever and wherever I do go.

* * *

1. What do you do to build a relationship with your medical personnel?
2. Do you know the nurses' names?
3. Have you ever gifted your doctor or nurse? Explain.

Do you acknowledge National Doctor Appreciation Day?

Developing a Relationship via Email

My chronic illness (Post-Polio syndrome) has not only given me more time to pray, but some unique ways to "meet people." In 2001, I had emailed one of our sports columnists about her prediction that our Miami Dolphins would win their game of the week. They did, and she was the only one, out of four, who had predicted the win. She responded to my email, and a friendly exchange began.

Early summer of 2002, I was in bed for four weeks, and she was in England covering Wimbledon. Our communication increased to almost daily messages. This led to our eventual face-to-face meeting over lunch. Since then I've been able to share my writing with her, congratulate her on her writing awards, and pray for her.

Without my extra time because of my illness, I probably wouldn't have the inclination or taken the time for this ongoing communication.

* * *

1. What relationships/friendships have you found since your illness/accident?
2. How did they develop or get initiated?
3. Do you have some other ideas that you'd still like to try?

Fatigue: The Life Robber

Toward the end of May, Ron and I stayed with our grandchildren, ages 9 and 11, and all was well until I played an innocent game of tossing two basketballs simultaneously among the four of us. You had to be quick so that you didn't end up holding two balls or getting hit by one before you passed the other one. It was great fun. The four of us were having a good time. We laughed when we forgot where to throw the ball next or ended up getting hit by an in-coming ball before getting rid of the first one.

But the next day it was no laughing matter when my body started screaming. O.K. I do have a bad knee that had a right to complain. And my arms and shoulders hurt—that was the voice of unused muscles speaking. But the fatigue—it rears its ugly head most days whether I'm active or not. And that day it demanded four naps!

I've learned that fatigue is a common factor for those of us with chronic conditions and/or injuries. And most days I've learned how to handle it—usually with two naps. But it's those days when its demands overshadow my plans that cause me to despair—to grieve for my former life of good health.

Before Post-Polio, I could and did plan multiple activities for one day and even more for the evening. My calendar was full to the brim. This person was a Type A in all caps. But whammo—I could no longer even plan one thing in the AM and another in the PM. I couldn't go out during the day and again at night. In fact, I try not to plan two activities on adjacent days now.

Fatigue: the guest that came to dinner and decided to become a permanent houseguest. It comes with a rest-ofyour-life warranty. Oh, we've all tried this supplement, that juice, this new Rx and even some things that we shouldn't have touched with a ten-foot pole, but fatigue is a reality in our lives.

Fatigue doesn't travel alone either—it brings relatives: moodiness, loss of socialization, weight gain, tempers, etc. We each have our own "cousins" that travel with fatigue. And we each must experiment and find our own coping mechanisms.

I've simplified my life. We've down-sized from 2,000 sq. ft. to 1200 sq. ft. That has made a big difference not only in my fatigue, but in my hip and knee. I also take naps and drink green tea. One polio doctor who spoke to our support group suggested that naps should be at least twenty minutes long; we should really rest—not watch TV or read a book, and if we have music on—it shouldn't have any words. This advice has helped me, and for what it's worth, I pass it on to you.

* * *

1. How do you cope with your fatigue?
2. Does your family understand your fatigue?
3. How do you handle advice from well-meaning people who want "to heal" you?

Less Stress, More Energy
Alternative Treatments

When I was working fulltime and felt like I could afford it, I started getting a massage every other week. For me, it became the greatest stress reducer. I eagerly looked forward to it and bemoaned the week I went without one.

But when my health began to change because of Post-Polio syndrome, I had to quit my job, and due to economics, the massages had to go. Without my massages, I began looking for ways to increase my energy. I started taking Co-Q 10, B-6, B-12, Vitamin E, and eating more protein and less "white" carbohydrates. This all helped.

My sore muscles from stress, leg cramps and knee pain from overused muscles, and new muscle weakness threatened to wreak more havoc with my energy. Then we bought a hot tub. It was a wonderful relaxer/DE stressor for my entire body.

But I still craved more energy. I was taking two to five naps a day. My thoughts returned to massage therapy. My doctor wrote a Rx for therapeutic massage, and our medical reimbursement program covered the cost.

Now I look forward to my visits from Diana. She brings her table to my home, spends an hour working me over, invigorating not only my muscles but my attitude also.

My chiropractor friend, Dr. Royce Newman, explained it to me this way: The muscle loss and new muscle weakness of Post-Polio has slowed down my physical activity, which in turn has slowed down my entire lymphatic system. It is no longer able to move all the bad toxins out of my body. The massage gets everything moving and, on their way, out. By the time Diana's done working on me, all fluids (toxins) are racing for an easy exit. This is why she always encourages me to drink plenty of water after a massage.

August of 2003, as we started on a road trip, I became so ill that I was laid out in the back seat with stomach cramps. We stopped at a friend's place and knew that we'd have to stay at least an extra day until I was well enough to travel. They, wisely, offered to make an appointment for me to visit their massage therapist.

The next day she gave me a deep massage, even my stomach. I returned to my friend's place, took a nap, got up and vomited, and felt like new. The next day we were able to continue our travel.

My doctor friend explained that it was the perfect example of my body's inability to rid itself of harmful toxins. (I had eaten pork, and it did not agree with me.) He went on to say that it was also the perfect example of the healthful benefits of massage.

That experience taught me a good lesson about my body's limitations and what I need to do to compensate. I now have a standing appointment every two weeks! Gwen now cares for me where we winter in Florida. When we moved to Tennessee, I immediately sought out a massage therapist. Gail came to our log cabin home every two weeks. What a dear friend she became!

* * *

1. Are you currently using any alternative medical treatments?
    Describe them.
2. What have been the results?
3. Do you recommend this to others?

My Church Was Too Fragrant

Perfume. Perfume everywhere, and not a breath of fresh air to be found. If someone, wearing a heavy scent, sat beside me, in front of me, or behind me, I'd have to get up and move. If I had a chance, I'd explain why. However, my explanation wasn't always appreciated.

At times, it'd take three or four moves before I'd find a "safe" spot. (Our sanctuary held 2,000 people.) After months of playing musical chairs because of the fragrance wearers, I gave up, and we moved to the balcony.

One would think that this was a solution, but the first row of the balcony was the "catching place" for the up-draft of perfumes from the congregation below. Finally, I found one row—midway in the balcony—that was O.K. The walkthru was directly in front of it, and the people who usually sat on the pew behind were generally the non-perfumed.

However, we left Sunday morning church the week that our church added a Saturday evening service. I was a happy congregant. People who attend Saturday services generally dress casually and don't take the time to douse with fragrances. Also, the service was moved to our new fellowship hall that didn't have a build-up of cleaning chemicals.

My contentment lasted three years until October 3, 2003, when Saturday night service was canceled until a new senior pastor was called. Where did this leave me? Unfortunately, I came down with the flu and was laid up for four weeks—choosing a church service became a non-issue.

Then we took a cruise for a week, and the holidays and some travel followed.

I had mentioned my difficulty to our administrative pastor a year before, but he didn't see it as a problem. However, I do know that choir members are told not to wear perfume. I wasn't ready to become a Sunday, TVchurch member either. My husband and I prayed for a long-term solution.

For us that solution did mean changing churches. And in God's all-knowing wisdom, this solution has brought with it many additional benefits.

* * *

1. What problems have you encountered with the greater community because of your health?
2. What have you done about it?
3. What advice do you give others about similar problems?

The Glass is Half-Full!

Humor me just for a minute and think about some of the good things that have happened since your injury, illness or life-changing event. Think of things and/or people that wouldn't have come into your life otherwise. Most of us don't have to ponder too long or too hard to come up with at least a short list.

Being carried out from work on a stretcher with symptoms of a heart attack was the beginning of the end for me. Even though it turned out to be stress, the damage to an already weakened body was done. I had to quit work. It seemed like the end of the world.

Since the onset of my Post-Polio syndrome or "polio crash" as some call it, my life has completely turned around. I used to teach writing, but now I am a writer. I used to tell people how to do it, and now I get to do it myself. It all started as a constructive, time-filling idea of a cheap Christmas present for my immediate family.

I gathered a few articles that I'd written—an old journal from time in Africa, and even my husband's love letters. Believe it or not, the articles sort of fell into categories, which became chapters, which became a book—a book of memories for my family for Christmas. My sons were so pleased that they read it straight through the day/night they received it.

There's no way that I would have had the time or the incentive to do this before I had to quit working.

And that was just the beginning. Since then I've written six books. I've found something that doesn't require an 8 to 5 commitment, but I can do it when and if I feel like it. I can even set it aside for months, and no one knows or cares. It's brought a new kind of fulfillment to me. I've discovered a creativity in myself that I used to bring out of others.

When someone tells me that they enjoy my writing because it brings back memories of their life or encourages them, I'm fulfilled. This probably wouldn't have happened if I were still working. And you know what, I'm so glad I get to do this! I'm not even sure that the glass is half-full anymore; it seems to be creeping more towards the ¾ mark.

* * *

1. List three things/activities or people that have enriched your life since your injury or illness that you wouldn't have met otherwise.
2. Write down three things that you do well.
3. Write five things that you like about yourself.

When Did It Become an Effort to Socialize?

We're experiencing the best weather we've had in a long time. Day in and day out the temperatures are in the high seventies or mid-eighties and there's always a nice breeze to cool a person and keep the bugs away. The farmers are complaining as they always do regardless, that we haven't had enough rain. They got their corn and soybeans in by last week and now I guess they have a legitimate concern over the lack of moisture.

I have coffee almost every morning with a group of professors that I used to teach with and lately we're having difficulty on deciding where the new site should be. Our old site in downtown Normal is virtually inaccessible because of all the building there in what is referred to now as "Uptown Normal." Fortunately for me, one of the possibilities is a new ice cream and coffee cafe three blocks from our house so I'm able to wheel over there and get my exercise to boot.

--R.A.

You have no idea how much I'm enjoying the give and take of this Internet exchange. It's so much easier to sit at the computer and share some pleasantries than it is to make the effort to leave the house and meet someone in person. I don't have to look good, and I don't even have to feel good.

The in-person connection is exciting and invigorating, but it leaves me drained. When did "having to be nice" become work? It seems like the simple give and take, in person, just drains me. Going to church and being with so many people is not easy for me any more either.

But our small group (probably like the coffee group above) on Thursday evening is just right—6 to 8 people.
We wear our casual clothes; we know everyone's name and background. We're comfortable. I don't have to explain, again, that the leg brace is because of Post-
Polio, which follows polio, etc., or that I'm having a shitty day.

Keeping social connections is especially vital for us. We need to keep our social selves alive to encourage our physical selves. And the friends we surround ourselves with need to be positive people.

I've found a couple of friendships that I just had to drop. One was always complaining and negative. Toxic. I didn't want to fall into her way of thinking. The other one was too controlling—it always had to be her choice of what we did. That can become demeaning when our viewpoint/input doesn't count. In fact, after I shared a few of her phone messages with a psychologist friend, he advised me to never see her again.

Friendship is vital. Social contact is important. At times we have to find alternative ways of maintaining them or become more selective with whom we share our meager amounts of energy.

* * *

1.   In what social setting are you most comfortable?
2.   Do you need to make any changes in your friendships?
3.   Do you need to socialize more? How could you do that?

Profiles of
Polio Survivors

Coming Down from the Mountain
Bruce E. Sachs

I first started to climb the mountain in August 1940 when as a 13-month-old boy I became stricken with polio. My family lived in Baraga, a small town about 75 miles from the only major hospital in the Upper Peninsula, which was in Marquette, Michigan. Being the youngest of three children, my parents were unable to stay in the area and were only able to visit me infrequently. I do remember hearing later that when my mother came to visit I called her, Mrs. Sachs, but when my dad came to visit I called him, Dad. I really didn't know family love until I was about two years old. The hospital had numerous polio patients that summer, with many of us being confined to iron lungs. I was confined to an iron lung constructed from an oil drum.

After spending about nine months in the hospital, I continued my climb up the mountain by learning to walk. With my right leg shorter than my left, and both arms affected, I learned to walk with the aid of a built-up shoe and a long leg brace. Although I could go home, my parents spent countless hours with my therapy. As I grew older, I detected that my brother resented the attention I received, but my sister became my supporter and my helper.

For the next few years, I continued my climb up the mountain by trying to be normal. I grew up in a small town with no handicapped education classes; therefore, I was encouraged to do everything the other children did. I played baseball, went fishing, walked my dog, and tried to be as good as I could at everything. My dad taught me all the outdoor activities, and my parents encouraged me to do whatever I could, with few restrictions.

Between the ages of 10-14, I returned to the hospital each summer for surgery on my right leg and left arm. Usually these stays consisted of 6-8 weeks of recovery and therapy. Again, my parents came to visit on an infrequent basis. Although the surgeries were of minimal help, I was able to discard my leg brace, and I continued to climb the mountain.

My parents moved to Wakefield, Michigan, another small town, before I started 8th grade. As with my previous school there were no handicapped education classes, so I continued in the general education classes. In high school I was unable to participate in sports, so I became involved in activities that did not require physical strength. One such activity was the Future Teachers of America Club, which led to my life's work as a schoolteacher. Several of my teachers encouraged me to become a teacher, and my brother, who graduated from college my senior year, introduced me to several friends that were becoming elementary teachers.

After high school, I again found myself in Marquette, but this time I was a student at Northern Michigan University. Along with my studies, I was a four-year member of Alpha Phi Omega, a National Service Fraternity, where I received an Outstanding Member Award my senior year. I also worked as an Assistant Boy Scout Master with a local troop.

After finishing college with an Elementary Teaching Certificate and a Master's Degree in Educational Leadership, I continued my climb. I moved to the Detroit area and then to Livonia. I was an elementary school teacher for 42 years, married, with one daughter.

This climb continued until about 1998, which was about 58 years after I had polio. At that time, I experienced sudden weakness in my right arm, which was my good arm. I continued to work, but for the first time in my life, I had to ask for help from my colleagues. Although there were no formal accommodations made for me, I did move my parking place closer to the building, and the staff started helping me with a variety of daily activities. I had always been independent and although the help was appreciated, I had to learn to adjust to my new condition. I had to start to "Come Down from the Mountain."

My wife died in 2002 and I retired in 2003. I started to follow the Post-Polio precept "conserve to preserve". I changed my focus from putting teaching first to putting my well-being first. I had much less stress, and I used my energy to continue my daily activities.

Being a true "type A" person, it has not been easy coming down the mountain. I can only hope that I have reached a plateau and can continue to help those around me. I have joined a retired school personnel group and recently have become a greeter at the

Since my retirement in June 2003, I have continued to be a greeter at the Post-Polio Clinic in Warren, Michigan, a co-facilitator of the Southeast Michigan Post-Polio Support Group, and I serve as Chairman of the Michigan Polio Network. I met my wife at my local support group.
Dianne is also a polio survivor, and we married in 2008.

We have participated, the last eleven Septembers in the "Post-Polio Wellness Retreat" at Bay Cliff Health Camp, Big Bay, Michigan. We have also attended several International Post-Polio Conferences. Although Post-Polio syndrome continued to affect my physical well-being, I continue to slowly "Come Down from the

Mountain".

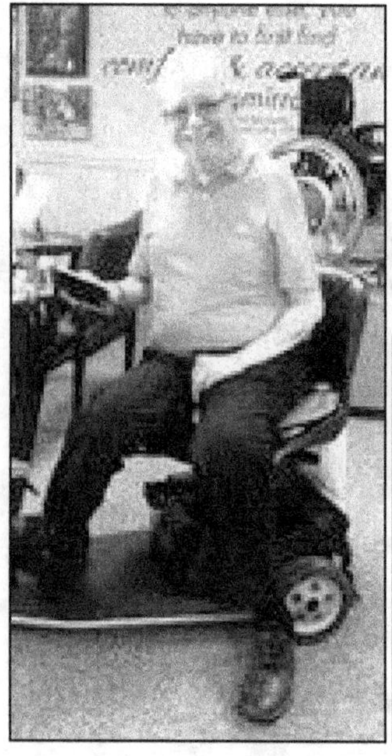

Bruce 2018

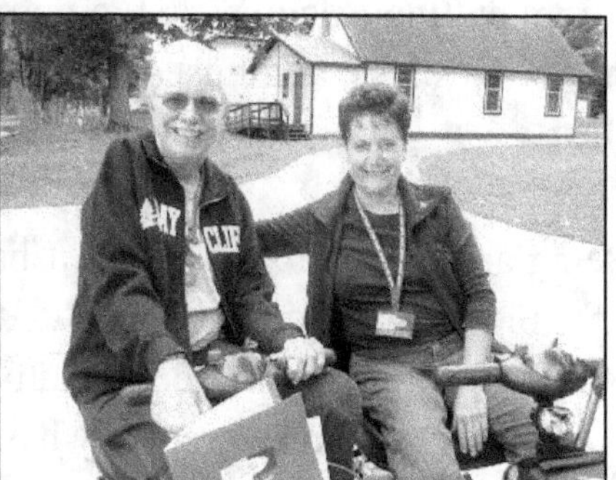

Bruce and Dianne

Back Then, The Wooden Lung
Fighting polio with boxes and vacuum cleaners
by Becky Kratz

In August of 1940, twenty-year old John Woods was vacationing in Grand Marais, hundreds of miles away from his home in Detroit. What started as a pleasant visit to the Upper Peninsula turned into a race against time when Woods was stricken with infantile paralysis, commonly referred to as polio.

He was transported down the length of Michigan by boat, airplane, and ambulance in search of an available iron lung—a large cylindrical machine that allows a person to breathe when their normal muscle control has been lost. The polio epidemic had taken hold of the U.P. at this time; within days, ninety cases were rushed to St. Luke's Hospital (now Marquette General). At least twenty-three of these cases had respiratory involvement and required the aid of an iron lung if they were going to survive.

Unfortunately, area hospitals were not ready for this kind of emergency. Woods and many other patients died before an unoccupied iron lung could be located.

St. Luke's only had one lung on hand when the influx of sick children poured through their doors during the fall of 1940, which had been purchased only weeks before as a "precautionary measure" when more and more cases of polio began to surface.

It was the only iron lung in the U.P. when the epidemic struck.

The staff of St. Luke's knew that the hospital was in over its head. With hospitals in Iron Mountain, Newberry and other surrounding cities in the same bind, they needed help; and they knew just the man to do it.

Maxwell K. Reynolds, a Princeton University graduate in engineering, had come to Marquette as a civil engineer with an explosives company. His passion for boating led to the founding of the Lake Superior Yacht Yard, and with it, the shop that would save the lives of at least nineteen polio-stricken children.

Reynolds responded to the call from the St. Luke's superintendent immediately, saying that he would fashion a device that could serve as a makeshift iron lung. He and his crew of eight mechanical and electrical engineers, carpenters, cabinet makers and tinsmiths first inspected the iron lung in use at St. Luke's, then began work on a homemade respirator from scratch.

"He went quickly to the old railway station and found an old refrigerator box, made of plywood in those days," recalled his grandson, Peter Frazier of Marquette. "He got that to the shop, and the crew started putting together the unit that I still have…he was a very inventive and creative person."

Construction on the wooden lung began at 3:30 p.m., and by 6:45 p.m. the same evening it was finished. It was five feet long and four feet wide with two and a half feet of depth, and was made air-tight with sponge rubber gaskets.

The vacuum effect needed to make the device work came from the home vacuum cleaner of Max's wife, Frances. A manually-operated vacuum release valve kept the lung going; the fast-fading health of the children left no time to upgrade the valve to operate automatically until later. The total cost to construct the lung was estimated at less than $40; $24 for labor and $10 for material.

A short time after the wooden lung was completed, a child suffering from respiratory paralysis was placed into it.
St. Luke's reported that the device was a success, and Reynolds and his crew worked day and night to create more of them out of oil drums, stove bolts, suction pumps, and anything else they could find, Frazier said.

Frances Reynolds assisted her husband by handoperating some of the first models that were not yet automatic, and their son Ted left his job in Wisconsin for a time to help build the lungs. With the support of his family, Max and the boating house crew ended up providing St.
Luke's with enough facilities to hold ten polio patients.

Although the fight to combat polio was a little less onesided than before, the illness hadn't yet run its course. A September 14, 1940 article from The Mining Journal states that, "Although continued improvement in the infantile paralysis situation has been noted in various parts of the
Upper Peninsula during the last two days...several additional cases have been received at St. Luke's Hospital."

With the help of Infantile Paralysis Foundation funds, St. Luke's was able to purchase additional factory-made iron lungs. That same year, the Mining Journal announced "stag" dinners that were held to fundraise for the purchase of an $1,850 iron lung for the Iron Mountain General Hospital that was used on a rental basis.

The polio epidemic left the U.P. in 1941, but its ravages were felt long afterwards. Of the 180 polio patients who passed through the Northern Michigan Children's Clinic and admitted to St. Luke's, 100 continued to receive orthopedic treatment at Bay Cliff Health Camp.

The residents of the U.P. did not soon forget the effects of the polio epidemic either. It is estimated that on the basis of population, the U.P.'s participation in the 1941 campaign for the National Infantile Paralysis Fund ranked high in the country, and that the total from that year's March of Dimes was the largest ever recorded from this region.

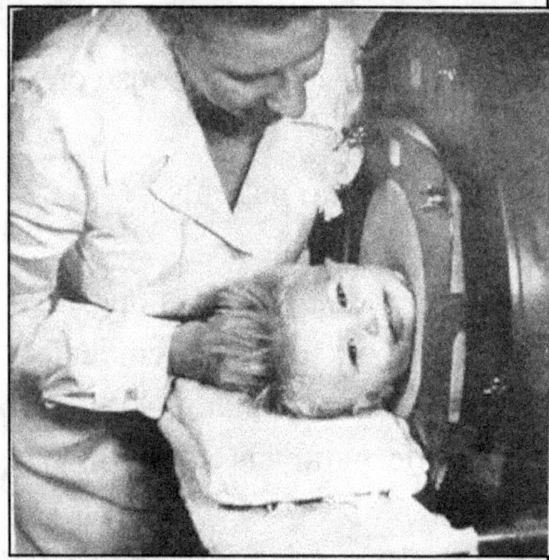

Bruce's picture was in the Dec 1940 Hygeia Magazine.
The caption reads:

"Ideas hashed through my mind like a neon sign. Respirators could be built but only hours were available for a task that needed days."
Here is a result of those flashes: a lung, and a life that was saved.

Twin Sisters Contract Polio
Become Poster Kids for March of Dimes & Easter Seals
Dianne Dych-Sachs

It was the summer of 1952. There was a large outbreak of polio that summer. There were three children in our family at that time. We lived in the Detroit area. My brother was 2 years-old, and he had a bad cold two weeks before my twin sister and I were stricken with polio at 13 months of age. My mother noticed that I would cry when she changed my diaper. This persisted along with the crankiness. My parents took me to the doctors, who recommended immediate hospitalization at Children's Hospital in Detroit where my polio virus was confirmed. The doctors asked if there were siblings at home. My sister was confirmed on a later date to have contracted a lighter case of polio.

My mother is a very strong woman, but she did cry when the doctor told her that her baby had polio, and that I would have to stay in the hospital. Later, I was transferred to Farmington's Children's Rehabilitation Hospital and given the Sister Kenny treatments. Being an infant, the nurses restricted movement by strapping me down with a cottonlike strap around my waist, tied to the crib.

Mom and Dad could not visit very often because of caring for my brother and sister, and Dad worked six days a week. However, my mother would call, and she remembers the nurses commenting on me being a good baby. Because I was so young when contracting polio, I have no memories of my hospitalizations. We were very fortunate the March of Dimes took care of all our medical bills.

After being released from the Rehabilitation Hospital, a physical therapist visited the house on a weekly basis. Debby and I were fitted with braces and amazingly learned to walk. When we moved to Macomb County, Easter Seals helped with our medical care. My sister and I became Poster Kids for the March of Dimes and later Easter Seals.

My parents treated my sister and me no different than our unaffected siblings. (Sister Laura was born four years after we had polio.) We had chores, responsibilities, and were always encouraged to do our best. If there was any teasing and our feelings were hurt, Mom explained to us that they were rude and didn't know any better. She also taught us never to feel sorry for ourselves, and that that there were people much worse off than us. Mom often said, "You can do anything in life that you put your mind to." I will always be grateful for those words.

One of my fondest childhood memories is attending handicap camp during the summer months. My sister and I attended Camp Grace Bentley located in Jeddo, Michigan. We were just seven years-old when we started attending camp, and we spent many summers there. I think it gave us a good perspective on life. We met many friends and still have kept in contact with some of the campers throughout all these years.

We attended regular school. It was initially recommended that we attend handicapped school. Mom would have nothing to do with that recommendation. She said there was nothing wrong with our minds, so off to regular school we went. We did just fine. We were not the first kids picked for team sports, and we were not the last. I missed most of my high school years, as I was homeschooled. I had five major surgeries on my right ankle trying to stabilize it so that I could walk without the brace. I was finally able to get rid of the brace in my twenties.

I had five major surgeries on my right ankle trying to stabilize it so that I could walk without the brace. I was finally able to get rid of the brace in my twenties. Debby and I both attended college and made the Dean's list. I ended up with an associate degree. I worked at a local hospital for 30 years as a Neuro/Vascular Technologist and later as a department supervisor. We both married and have lovely families. I have been blessed with many grandchildren to love.

About ten years ago, Post-Polio arrived. It is very hard to slow down when my brain is telling me differently. I did have to go on disability in 1998. I am back in braces and using a cane. I have a scooter-friend that definitely conserves energy. I keep busy with our local Polio support group. I am secretary and board member of the Michigan Polio Network, and I volunteer as a greeter at St. John's Polio Clinic in Warren, Michigan.

My husband Bruce is also a polio survivor. We have discovered this wonderful place called Bay Cliff Health Camp located in Big Bay, Michigan. We have met other polio survivors at this wellness camp and look forward to the event in the fall

My sister hasn't done so well. She developed Multiple Sclerosis many years ago. She has maintained a positive attitude through all this. She is legally blind and confined to a wheelchair most of the time. However, she is still able to make beautiful greeting cards.

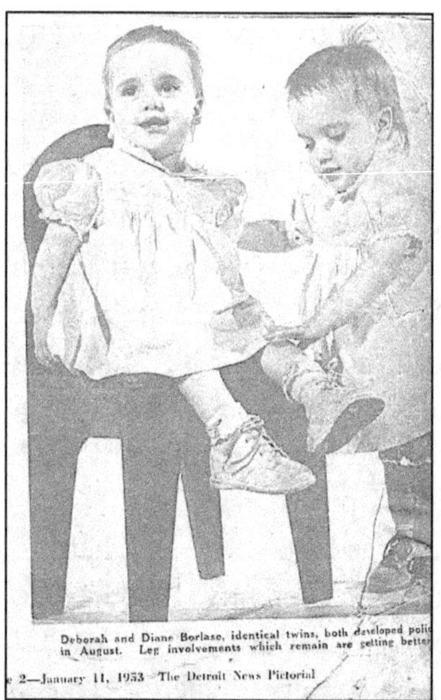

Deborah and Diane Borlase, identical twins, both developed polio in August. Leg involvements which remain are getting better.

2—January 11, 1953—The Detroit News Pictorial

Deborah and
Diane Borlase,
identical twins,
both developed
polio in August.
Leg involvements
which remain are
getting better.
January 11,
1953
The Detroit
News Pictorial

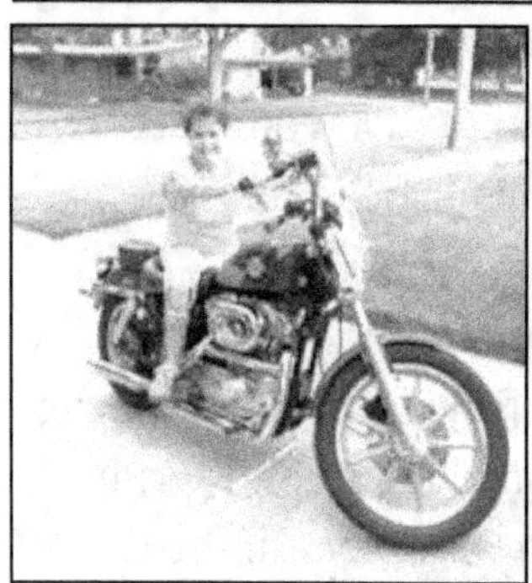

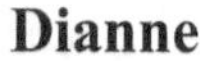

Dianne

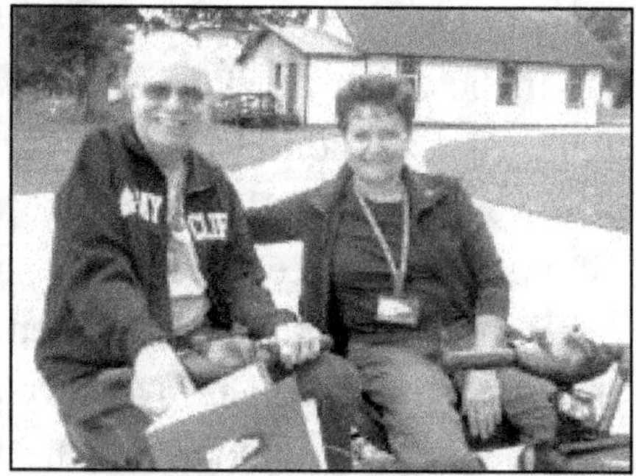

Bruce and Dianne

Polio: First the Bad, Then the Good
Phyllis Porter Dolislager

1944, while living in Greenville, Michigan I contracted polio. I was 18 months old. They guessed that I might have gotten it from the lake water, because the family had spent a lot of time at the local lakes that summer.

The first sign Mother noticed was that I walked with a limp. She took me to see their family doctor, Marco Hansen, and he referred us to a specialist in Grand Rapids. But that doctor told her to take her daughter home—she had only bumped her leg! Apparently, polio was on the minds of all the mothers, and for any slight problem they were having their children examined.

Time went on, and one day I fell—my leg could no longer hold me. This time Mother took me to a polio specialist at Blodgett Hospital, and it was confirmed: Polio. Darcy and Eleanor (mother and father) carried me around from approximately the age of two to four. I did get a leg brace before starting kindergarten. One time we stopped at Ramona Park on the way home from seeing the doctor. I wanted to ride the merry-go-round, but it wasn't open. When the man saw my brace, he started the hand-painted, wooden horses going just for me and gave me the longest ride ever!

During this time, I had to lie in bed with my foot in a box so that the sheet wouldn't touch my polio foot. Apparently, this theory went along with not wanting me to put any weight on my foot. I remember lying flat on my back, watching a spiral-cut piece of paper placed on a stick on the heat register, spin around. George, the farmhand, made that to entertain me.

My polio befell the family before they were farmers. A pivotal decision coincided with the onset of full-time farming. Dad and Mother went to see the Sister Kinney movie. It illustrated a new method of treating polio patients. It advocated muscle massage to reactivate the lost muscles, rather than the bracing that took over for the muscles and caused them to atrophy. About this same time, Dr. Louis Dobbin opened his chiropractic office in Rockford. He said he would work with me if they'd take my leg brace off. This was a weighty, but consequential decision to make. They knew that after having to carry me everywhere for two years, the leg brace had allowed me to finally walk on my own. Yet future years without having to wear the leg brace sounded good too. In 1947, they made the decision to take the brace off.

Mother took me to Dr. Dobben for therapy on my leg three times a week for two years, and then two times a week for four years. Surely the income of a new farmer was stretched to provide this treatment, but it was rewarded. To this day I still walk without a leg brace, but I do wear a knee brace on my good leg. They always had to buy two pair of shoes because my feet had a difference of three shoe sizes; the shoes required extra construction on the inside also.

The summer between my 9th and 10th grades, I had corrective surgery on my foot. Dr. Caulkins, a partner of the doctor who originally told Mother to take her daughter home, that she had only bumped her leg, reshaped my foot with a procedure called a triple arthrodesis. I have had five other surgeries on my foot since that time. Buying two pair of shoes never changed, but I was finally able to wear shoes other than the orthopedic ones with special construction inside my polio/right shoe as my polio foot was misshapen.

Throughout this time my family never treated me any differently. I had chores to do like any other farm girl. My polio never held me back; the survivor mentality set in. I went to college: two years at Taylor University and two more years at Central Michigan University where I graduated with a BA in speech. Later I earned my MA from Michigan State University in curriculum and education, and I have taken post-graduate hours in English at Florida Atlantic University. Most of my life I have been an educator: speech, forensics, drama, journalism, literature, and writing. I directed plays, coached debate and forensics, and sponsored school newspapers, etc. My last position was as a writing adjunct professor at Nova University.

I met my husband while teaching at North Muskegon High School. I wondered if there would be any negative reactions from Ron toward my physical problem. Imagine my surprise to learn that his sister, Lois, had polio when she was six; Lois was a quadriplegic.

In the late 60's, through the NOSE (National Odd Shoe Exchange), I began exchanging shoes with a gal in Minnesota whose feet were the exact opposite of mine!
Although we never met, it continued until she passed away.

Post-Polio took me out of the classroom in 2001. After I sent a letter to the governor of Florida, Jeb Bush, I was granted social security disability. I refused to pay a lawyer to help me through the process. That's my Type A, post-survivor mentality.

About this same time, Ron and I visited our lawyer to update our will. I walked into the lawyer's office with a duty to perform—update our will. But I walked out with a new purpose for living. I walked in a polio survivor who had to quit teaching my writing classes because of a plethora of physical problems. But I walked out with a writing assignment.

As the lawyer completed the necessary paperwork that day, she told us about the "missing part" of our will: our testament. Of course, I'd heard the phrase, "Last Will and Testament", but I hadn't given it much thought until then. I thought of a will as a legal document intended to divide up one's property and to provide for one's heirs. However, I learned that there is another kind of will that has been in use in the Judeo-Christian traditions. It is the Last Will and Testament or an Ethical Will.

These wills are a kind of spiritual document. They are written in the belief that the wisdom and values acquired in a lifetime are as much a part of a family's legacy as are all its material possessions.

I don't think our lawyer had in mind a book when she presented the idea, but as a woman of faith, I'd experienced God's direction in my life over and over again. I had a lot to share. I was ready to write. Once again, I had a purpose in life—a goal.

As I was no longer working and not receiving a paycheck, I decided to write some of my family's stories as a Christmas gift for them. I thought, and I wrote throughout the year. When December came, I had a book to give our sons. (We copied it at home and bound it.) They were so pleased that they stayed up all night and read all 125 pages.

My plan was to share my "Testament," my book, with our families only. But almost immediately others wanted to read it. We ended up doing three printings. Then it was published by Xulon Press and made available on Amazon. Soon I began giving workshops, encouraging others to write their stories also. Oh boy, I was teaching again!

As I reread my own book, *A King-Size Bed, A Silk Tree, and a Fry Pan,* I was blessed to read—in print—how God's hand had been on my life. I wept many tears as I experienced anew His love through the rereading of those events. What had started as a gift for my family, proved to be a wondrous gift of remembrance for me, also. And . . . the motivation to continue writing.

I now have written ten books. Not bad for something that started out as a routine visit to the lawyer's office to update a will. Not bad for a person who was mourning the loss of her health and her career. Who says that "good" can't come out of "bad"? Not me.

At that time, I was using a power chair most of the time. Then I gained some weight, and I got beyond the overwhelming fatigue and depression. I started walking more, using a cane. After a recent trip and fall, I started using a walker at home and while grocery shopping. I do most of my other shopping online.

To date, I have published 10 books since Post-Polio hit me.

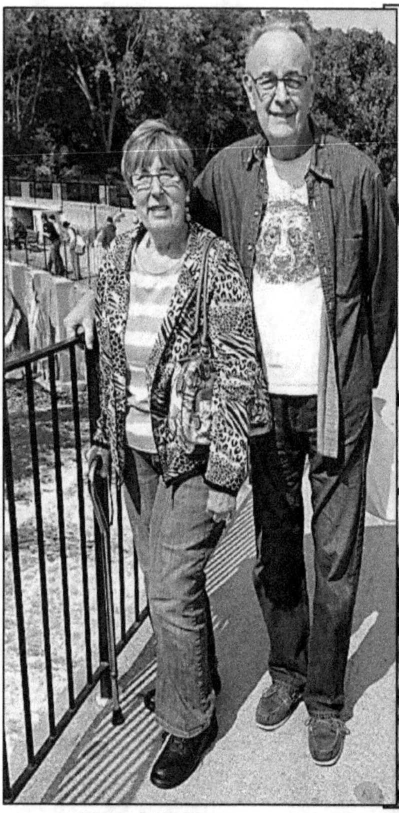

Phyllis with cane and Ron 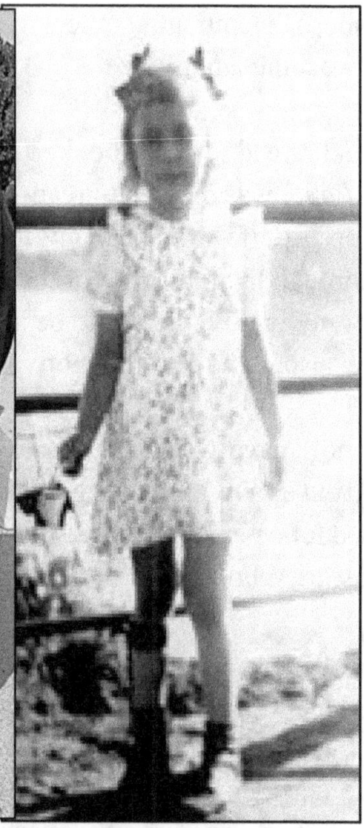   **Phyllis with br ace**

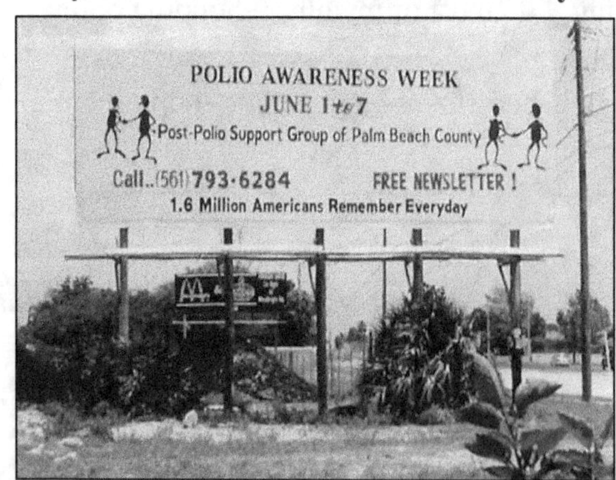

Billboard
designed
by Phyllis

She Can Get Up by Herself
Maureen Sinkule

I was born in 1951in Bay Ridge, Brooklyn, NY, and I had an older brother David, age 3, Sadly, I never sat my parents down to get the whole story. This is what I was told and what I remember:

On November 11, 1953, at age two, I was running a temperature. My neck hurt, and my grandmother noticed that I was tripping each time I walked, I was taken to a hospital by taxi, as my brother David remembers, He peeked into the examining room where he witnessed a doctor putting something down my throat, I was diagnosed with polio, hospitalized, and my immediate family was quarantined, The doctors told my mother to stay away from me because Polio was so contagious, but she held me even tighter.

Two days after I contracted Polio, was my brother's 5th birthday, and he was running around saying, "Where's my party, where's my party?" In sympathy, and even though in quarantine, one of my great aunts visiting from Egypt walked to the store and brought back party goods and made a party for him! As a result, my great aunts were quarantined and had a three-month delay back to Egypt and Lebanon because of the contagious nature of the epidemic.

Grandma was so upset that she cursed God for inflicting me with Polio, and about a month later [December 1953] when [King] David started coming down with the same symptoms, Grandma got down on her hands and knees and said, "Forgive me, forgive me – I accept Maureen, but not David, too!"

My mother told me that the March of Dimes said that if she gave me to them, they would pay for everything. Her response was, "They are not taking my daughter anywhere!"

My parents and my mother's sister's family purchased a two-family house in 1954, that only had one step to enter. At that time, I started to stutter because my brother always answered first, not giving me a chance. So, he was sent to sleep-away camp, giving my
stuttering a chance to subside,

For the next year, Mom carried or pushed me in a stroller everywhere. One day her older cousin came over and said, "Gin, you can tell me to mind my own business, throw me out of your home, but you cannot carry Maureen for the rest of her life! I've made and paid
for an appointment with a doctor to see Maureen."

Home physical therapy of stretching my legs started and was costly, Dad was only making about $80 a month, so Mom asked and was taught, and she gave me PT on our kitchen table.

My dad took movies of me while at St. Charles Hospital on Hicks Street, Brooklyn. Christmastime, 1955, a famous baseball player and TV personality, Officer Joe Bolton came with gifts and to entertain the children. Most there had polio, Mom told me that I always wanted her to be the first in line for visiting, and she did her best to comply. I was not hospitalized for very long, nor did I have any surgery,

By 1956, I had been fitted with two, long leg-braces w/waist band, wooden crutches, and I learned to walk, sit, fall, do stairs, etc. through out-patient PT, For some reason, still etched in my brain was the daunting full flight of 15 steps I eventually graduated to in the hospital, The physical therapist wanted me to climb up, and I remember saying, "I can't," and I was encouraged until I made it all the way up and down the stairs!

Whenever my family went anywhere I was their 'pass' to not have to wait in line or 'Mom's love letter to the police'
– "Little girl on braces and crutches receiving PT or whatever – I must park here, Thank you, Mrs. Naman." Once she did get a parking ticket and proceeded to take me to court where the judge said, "Dismissed!"

In November 1958, my parents, brother, and I flew complimentary to CA as dad worked for American Airlines, On the plane over, Charles Laughton and Elsa Lanchester befriended us and gave my family a ride in their limo to the
Hotel Roosevelt, in L.A, He gave us a letter addressed to
"Dear Walt, Take care of my friends."

Mom and Dad did everything possible to have me lead a normal, independent life, including school. Mom once told me that I did not go to a "special" school because I didn't live in a "special" world.

I made my first Communion, May 16, 1959, and Grandpa, being a shoe manufacturer, made my ugly brown, high-top shoes white, and my dad, with my brother's help, used contact paper to make my crutches white. We had a great celebration, despite the fact that my braces broke later that day and proved to be the beginning of many more breaks!

Sometimes I'd fall in church, and Mom would stop people from helping me saying, "She can get back up all by herself."

They thought the worst of her for it. Years later, Mom was approached by those same people, after seeing me as an adult, and they now understood and applauded her for making me independent.

In the summer of 1960, I was 9 years-old and sent to camp for children with disabilities, Surprisingly, we slept in tents raised 18 inches off the ground, I remember asking for assistance and was told, "You can do it." I proceeded to and fell, breaking my left arm. My dad came and took me to a hospital. I had a cast put on and spent the rest of the summer at St. Charles Hospital, until my cast came off as I was unable to walk using my crutches. While there, I met other children with polio, who had various types of rehabilitative surgery. One little boy had no limbs – a victim of Thalidomide, Then Hurricane Donna blew in! My classmates wrote me in the hospital about the downed trees and what they were doing in school.

In 1965 and 1967, I had bilateral ankle surgeries, enabling me to get rid of my right brace, I had my first job in 1967 and also volunteered at the VA Hospital for a few summers taking three buses to get there. To this day, I have always worn a left, long-leg brace, forearm crutches, and in 1999, I went to a short right brace when surgery failed,

I had and have the tendency to put weight on easily as I was not physically active and loved to eat! The doctor always told my mother, "If you love her, don't feed her."

In high school I took a Commercial Course, thinking that I'm not going to college, and the teachers would let me out five minutes early to get a head start to my next class, I was involved in activities including typing for the school paper, going to/helping out at dances and prom committee. I took hand-controlled driving lessons in 1969 and graduated high school in 1970, My high school guidance counselor had told me about NYS Vocational Rehab, who gave me the opportunity to go to college anywhere in the world,

I wanted to attend University of Miami, and because I did not have a math, science, or language, they suggested I first attend Miami Dade Community College, Kendall, FL, Voc Rehab provided tuition, books, and three-round trip flights home per year. I graduated and received an Associate in Science in Secretarial Science in 1972, I was never a
'student' and was very happy receiving my 2-year degree!

I stayed in Kendall and found a job as Office Manager in the Financial Aid Office at Miami Dade CC for the next 10 years, and I retired prior to my marriage in 1983, Matthew was my honeymoon baby born in 1984, and unfortunately, we divorced in 1987, I assisted in Sunday school for three year-olds and had odd, home-based jobs to supplement my income, I once attended a Miami polio support group in 1987, and after listening to everyone, I said to myself, I don't have any aches/pains – what am I doing here?!

One by one, my family began moving to Kendall. In 1993, Hurricane Andrew blew us up to Boca Raton, with my family following one at a time. My main job was raising Matthew and giving him the best education. I found Spanish River Church where I got involved in the Singles Ministry organizing plays/shows, activities, greeter for Sunday Bible study class and covered-dish parties. In 1999 and 2000, Matthew and I took two bus trips – five European countries, and we visited US National Parks. He pushed me all over in a manual wheelchair.

I met Carolyn DeMasi, and we started Boca Area Post-Polio Group in 1996, newsletter 1997, conference 2000, and annual cruises in 2003, At our February 2004 meeting, the Good Lord sent Joel to our support group.
He became my husband in October of that year,

I do not know if I ever have been diagnosed with PPS, In March 2016, Joel and I were involved in a 70mph head-on collision on I-95 fracturing my C2 and right femur, We have not been the same since, I do know that any type of trauma can have an adverse effect on us, Our used BraunAbility Toyota has been a blessing, I have not walked since April 2017—perhaps just being lazy, and I use a power chair full time.

Joel and I have 4 children/4 grandchildren. It has been a whirlwind adventure these past 14 years with our blended families. We enjoy family, friends, grandchildren, church activities, entertaining, yearly cruises, and taking care of each other.

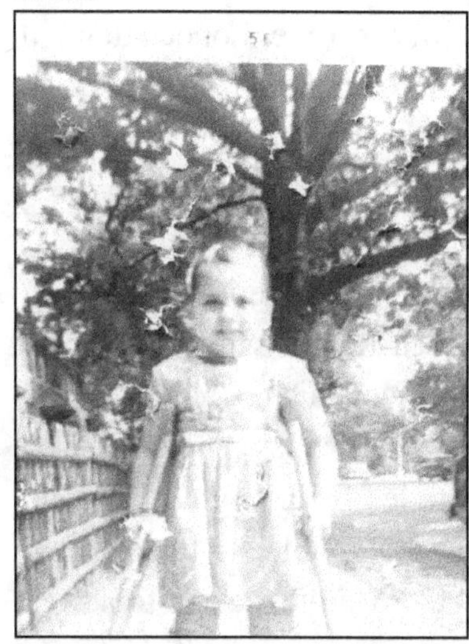

Maureen with crutches

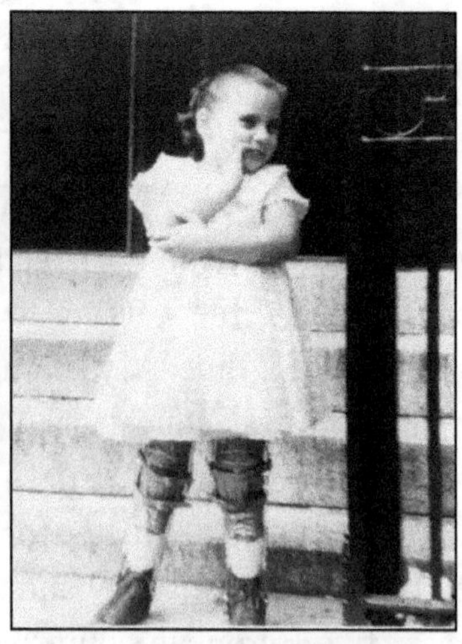

Maureen with Braces

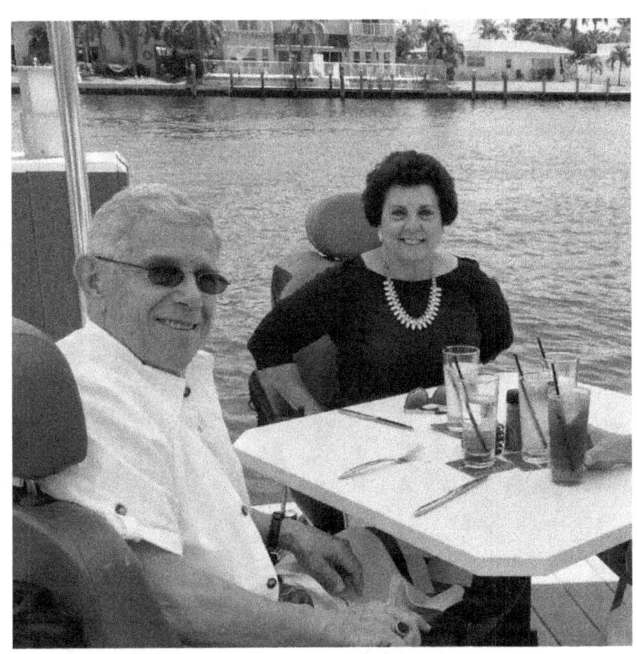

Joel and Maureen in power chairs

57

Eye of the Storm

Walking: The Magical Attraction

All of a sudden, I was lying on the
bathroom floor.
"Did you faint?" Ron asked.
I really didn't know.
But I did know that I was cold.

As he'd helped me out of the tub,
I'd put my weaker foot out first.
And as the rest of me followed . . . down I'd
gone.

Oh, the indignity to be crumbled
on the floor . . .
weak . . . faint . . . cold . . . wet.
I cried.

The leg cramps throughout the night had
foreshadowed this event.
And walking on the uneven ground at the
Spring Festival the evening before had
probably triggered the cramps.

It's back to the power chair or be
prepared to face more indignity.
It really shouldn't be such a difficult decision. But
walking has such a magical attraction once it's
been taken from us.

April 28, 2007

* * *

1.   What indignities have you had to face?
2.   How did you handle it?

Shopping While Sitting

It happened again. My leg gave out, and I had to grocery shop using my power chair. First of all, it's a pain in the butt to have to ask Ron to get the chair out of the car and to assemble it.

But the worst part is not being able to see or reach from a chair. Only one-third of the shelves are readable or accessible. This increases the shopping time.

Then there are the other shoppers . . . the ones who think you're taking up too much space or moving too slow. However, their response is much worse when I use one of the power carts that stores provide. Then people are just plain rude—as if I'm using it just for the free ride or something.

And speaking of those store carts, perhaps the worst part is the hideous—beep, beep, beep—it makes when you put it into reverse. How embarrassing! Perhaps that's one of the reasons that other customers give dirty looks to anyone using one.

But there is some good news buried in this muck. At least I have my own power chair and a willing husband to help me. And most of the produce is at eye level.

Oh yes, and that occasional meeting with another customer on wheels and the exchange of smiles reminds me that I'm not alone in facing life in a power chair. In fact, there's a whole community of us. We need to reach out to one another—to share the good and the bad—the victories and the challenges.

No, we're not alone. We're not the first ones to "do life on wheels." Now that's an encouraging thought right there!

* * *

1.   What activity outside the house presents a challenge to you?
2.   How do you handle it?
3.   Do you have any advice that you would give to others?

Is This the Time?

Suddenly, I don't want to be left alone.
I've always been strong and independent,
but now I've turned into a weeping wimp.
Why do feelings of weakness bring tears?

Is this just a cycle that I'm going through?
Will my strength and emotions once again plateau?
Or is this the time—the time that it's for real?
Is this the time that my energy doesn't return?

My fear has almost immobilized me.
It's making me cling to my husband,
not wanting him to travel next week.
It's put my mind through countless scenarios.

Will I be strong enough to accept new weakness?
Will my friends stick by me?
Will I have to give up all my work?
Is God asking me to rely on Him more?

Is this the time that I put feet to my faith?
Or is this the time that I wait patiently for God?

Be merciful to me, O God, Be merciful to me!
For my soul trusts in You;
And in the shadow of Your wings
I will make my refuge. (Psalm 57:1)

Thoughts of Despair

Life is looking downward into a vortex
spinning counterclockwise.
Gone is the sun.
Gone are the blue skies.
Only gray, stormy clouds remain.

And this vortex is the sucking kind. As I
lean over to get a better look, it reaches up
trying to draw me in.

It brings dark thoughts to my mind.
Thoughts of wheelchairs and minivans and lifts.
Thoughts of no longer walking.
Thoughts of dependency and despair.

Where is God in all of this?
Is this His plan?
Would He stoop to this?
Can't He do better?
Doesn't He *need* me to be working?

Or is He trying to get my attention
focused on Him and His power? Is He
reminding me that
He'll never leave me nor forsake me?

Lord, help me to willingly embrace the
future that You have for me.

Help me to embrace You and Your
will for my life.
I know that You don't **need** me to
accomplish Your agenda.
But *I* need to be willing to accept
Your will for my life.

Amen and Amen
9/13/03

* * *

1. Have you faced days like this?
2. What are your fears?
3. How do you handle them?
4. Have you ever written about your experience? Give it a try.

Inspirational Thoughts

Contentment

The mountains don't complain; They
continue to pose for us.
No matter the season, no
matter the weather.

But I wonder . . .
Do they ever wish that they could jump rope? or
skip from cove to cove calling,
"you're it" to their nearest neighbor.

Or are they content to sit with their hands
folded in their laps— an inspiration to all
mankind who come to gaze on their
majesty?

Their silent beauty stretches before us proclaiming the
awesomeness of God.
Oh, that you and I could be more like the non-
complaining mountains.

5/07

* * *

1. What part of nature brings you peace?
2. How often do you get to experience it?
3. Would you get the same feeling from having a pet dog or cat?

Do Angels Drive Trucks?

Tom Vander Molen

It was a boxy looking 1972 Plymouth Valiant. It wasn't the kind of car a high school senior dreams of, but it was my own, gifted to me by a caring parent. It may have been humble looking, but it was fast, and it was my first taste of driving freedom. As a 17-year-old high school senior, I had just secured my long-coveted driver's license when a malignant tumor began pressing on the nerves in my lower spinal cord, silently changing things inside my body. Half my senior year was spent in and out of hospitals with surgery, radiation, and chemo . . . finally to embrace a paralysis that would be mine for life.

A gradual turn-around would come in those months of fear and pain. During a stay in a rehabilitation facility, I was shown other ways to ambulate and how to live the life I had been dealt, a first taste of paralysis. In rehab, I was shown how to use my arms to compensate for legs which could no longer move. I was shown how to sit up in bed, put on my own clothes, prepare my own meals, and at the end of all of it, how to get behind the wheel of a car (even my own Plymouth) and to drive again.

It took installing some mechanical hand controls, a steering knob, and an upside-down Coca-Cola crate on the rear floor to support the folding wheelchair I would stow there for each trip out. Oh, and there was a long rope attached to the passenger side door. Once entering that side, I would slide across the front seat, stash the chair in back, then pull shut that door with the rope – and then, at last to start up the engine and drive! That almost intoxicating sense of independence (following a long and arduous road to recovery) had returned.

And so, I drove. I drove to meet friends, drove to summer picnics, drove to church, drove to college classes. And often, on my way home from school on Friday evenings, I would take long, random, unhurried routes home, over long, winding country roads, chasing the setting sun, or even the rising stars.

On a crisp, dark, autumn night I once let my newfound sense of freedom get the best of me. I'd landed in an empty parking lot of a church somewhere far outside the city limits to take in a fresh view of the Milky Way. Then it was time to head home. I set out to loop back to one of the main roads, but the street I'd taken was getting me nowhere. I had to turn around, which meant using someone's driveway.

It was well after 10 PM, and I was far off the beaten path. The roads were paved there, but traffic had long silenced. And it was dark—so very dark. There was nothing but the occasional yard light or reflector to remind me where I need to be. I crept my way to an open driveway and positioned my 2-door sedan right up to it (best as I could see), and shifted into reverse. A little pull on the gas lever, and I crept a little more. . . until . . .THUD! My trusty auto was angling upward from the bottom of a ditch—a ditch I had no idea existed!

In the muted silence of a rural, Friday night, I was sitting comfortably in a car, which has been swallowed whole by a culvert trench. On instinct, I grabbed the door handle and tried opening the door. It moved an inch, straight into the soft grass. It, and I, could go nowhere. I couldn't signal anyone, in that age long before cell phones. I was, at that moment, truly alone.

Three thoughts surfaced in my mind: I have headlights and I can flash them, but it is not likely anyone will see them. I have a car horn and could blast it until someone comes (assuming anyone is home). Or, I could pray, asking God to somehow care enough for a trapped college student to send some form of help.

There should be a fourth thought in all of this, in that I should be panicking. But I wasn't. I was just still. And in that quiet stillness, I was drawn to a pair of headlights sweeping down the road, heading in my direction. This was almost too good to be true. It appeared that they saw me, and I do not reach for the horn button. I waited . . . for them, . . . but off they went.

Thinking it might be time to panic, the passing vehicle stopped, reverses, and slowly backs up to the ditch. They saw me! But ... who are "they?" What kind of people are stopping? There was little time to wonder.

From the vehicle (a pickup truck) emerges a tall, bearded young man, and a companion, a young woman, who is sipping from the crinkled mouth of a large paper bag.

"Heeyyy, there! Looks like you might need a little help," he says, into my now open car window.

We converse a little. I tell him that for just a split second's time, I got overconfident behind the wheel (or maybe just plain cocky?) and landed square in the ditch. "What do you suggest?" I ask, not at all sure of what they could do to help me.

"Well, I do a little towing, and I just happen to have a pull chain here, and a winch. Heh! We can have you out in no time," he says.

"I would be ... SO grateful," I tell them, stumbling even for the words to keep up with what's so quickly unfolding. As we exchange names and small talk, the bearded pickup truck driver hooks my car up, tells me to take the car out of gear, and the process begins. Up, up, up I go . . . to level ground on the road.

Overcome with relief and gratitude, I pulled out what little cash I had in my wallet, as a bit of tangible thanks for the man. He waves me off and tells me to just have a good night and a safe drive home. They drive off, still the only ones aside from me, on that lonely country avenue.

What just happened here? In less time than it would have taken me to even think through my situation, let alone panic over it, there had appeared a vehicle: a pickup truck, outfitted with towing gear, driven by a couple who "happened to see me" on a dark night, in a ditch, and they were intrigued enough to stop to help me.

As I carefully drove home, in the sudden silence that came over me, I worked through a long, stammering list of improbabilities: *I should still be in that ditch*, I thought. *It could have taken until sometime on Saturday for someone to see me in that ditch.*

To this day, I exhaust no time wondering whether those two rough-cut country dwellers were supernatural beings, appearing suddenly from another realm to help me that night. They weren't quite "angel types," after all.

They did, however, appear. They appeared to me, with just the right kind of hardware, and at just the right time to answer a prayer I had not quite even begun to utter. What I know is that I was helpless and alone, and that I was rescued from a very real pit, in the middle of almost nowhere, on a dark and quiet night.

And that the word "coincidence" falls short in my mind when I try to explain this simple story to those who may care to hear it.

* * * *

That moment (there in the ditch) I remember to this day as a time when I absolutely knew I was being watched over by God. The complexities of it are staggering to my mind. Angels are "messengers of God," as we know. These were more like "servants of God" with hands and feet (and truck) available to help.

It was just such a powerful reminder to me that even without the use of my legs, God was there with me in a distinct way in those early days while I learned the ropes of this new way of living.

The above is an excerpt from: *Angels on Duty,*
A Collection of Angel Encounters,
Available at Amazon.com

Tom at the time of story

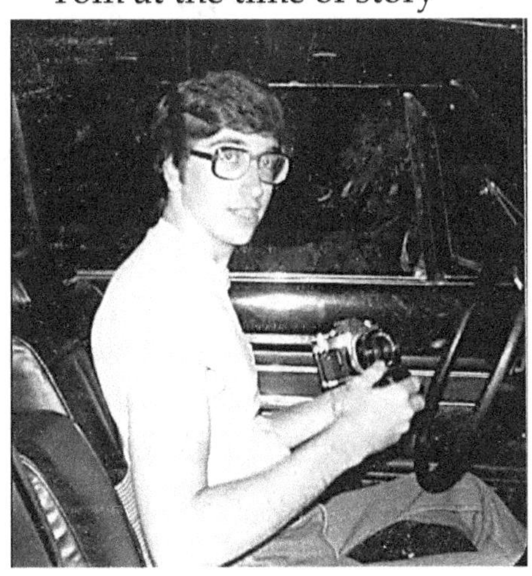

Tom today

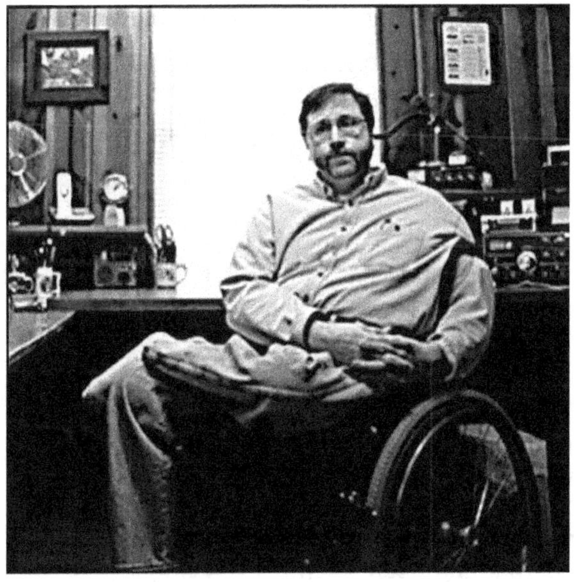

Reading . . . and Writing

Reading was a lifeline for me.
It's how my mother kept me lying flat
in bed when I had polio as a two-year old.
She read to me.

I learned all the nursery rhymes,
and all the fairy tales.
When I finished kindergarten,
I was promoted to second grade.

Then the book mobile came to our country school,
and I was reading for myself.
I devoured the Little House on the Prairie books.
Our family subscribed to the daily newspaper,
and I anticipated
each new installment of Uncle Wiggly.

In church, I shifted gears,
and I learned to read the Bible.

Then it was on to high school
and more intense reading and writing.
I worked as an aide in the high school library.

Would I ever have made it to college without my love
of reading that had been so finely developed?

When I became a high school teacher,
I read love letters from my future husband, Ron.
I knew I was going to marry him at our first meeting,
but I fell in love with him from reading his letters.

And the cycle of reading continued
as we read to our sons, Fred and Tom.

Now, I not only continue to read,
but I also write.
Perhaps it's only fitting that my most-read book is
Lessons Learned on the Farm
where reading began for me.

Dreams Can Become Realities

It was one of those firsts in my life. Our older son (wise age of 39) sat me (wise age of 60ish) down and asked me just how much thought had gone into my desire to leave a condo in sunny South Florida and buy a log cabin in the Smoky Mountains. Of course, he and I both knew the answer to that: None . . . Zero . . . Zip.

Until that beautiful April day, enhanced by the spring blooms of Tennessee's dogwood and red buds, I had envisioned Ron and me retiring in a condo with little maintenance. That was before our daughter-in-law, and I had toured some overpriced, under-designed condos on a lake and a golf course.

The following day Fred and I visited some condo complexes in the city of Knoxville. They may have been more in our price range, but not one of them held any promise for a wheelchair user. All our hopes seemed to have gone askew until I started looking through a local real estate magazine, and my eye zeroed in on a log cabin with the caption, Handicap Accessible.

Fred and I, and our realtor, Ina Painter, headed east to Townsend, one of the entrances to the Great Smoky Mountain National Park. After following a winding road, up and down and around, we saw it: A perfect, 1200 sq. ft., 2-bedroom, 2-bath, log cabin in the mountains . . . without any steps!

After I'd been inside about two minutes and had inhaled the knotty pine fragrance and checked out the fireplace, I announced, "We'll take it." Of course, neither Ina nor Fred paid any attention to me; they continued looking around, so I followed them.

Fred took lots of photos with his digital camera for Ron. I finally came to my senses and decided that I wasn't going to buy our retirement place without Ron. (Give me some credit, Fred.) But to my defense, Ron fell in love with the log cabin just from the photos.

Two weeks later we both returned, looked at a couple of other cabins for price comparison, and made our offer. (Of course, all the others had steps and none of them were brand new like ours.) The builder, Matt Kobolak, had purposely built the cabin to be accessible or easily converted to be. He was thinking ahead to the boomer population getting ready for retirement and that very few cabins on the local rental programs are accessible.

The cabin has wide, 36" doorways, a Jacuzzi tub and a freestanding shower in each bathroom. The closets are walk-in or roll-in. The clothes rods could be put at any height. Even the door to the back deck is 36" wide and accommodating, and the doors all have lever handles instead of knobs. The driveway and entrance were paved for the wheelchair.

The only thing missing in our cabin was the use of rocker switches instead of typical light switches. More and more builders around the country are using Universal Design as they build.

Selling our 2,000 sq. ft. house and moving to an 1150 sq. ft. condo in 2005 was our transition into downsizing and soon to be retirement living. Fewer steps immediately made a difference for me with my Post-Polio. I had been using my power chair almost full time in our larger home. Now when my leg gives out, I can easily use my power chair.

Thank goodness, "Handicap Accessible" is becoming more and more available. Don't limit yourself. Be aware. Look for a builder and/or a realtor who will listen to and accommodate your needs. The options are out there, but it's up to us to discover them.

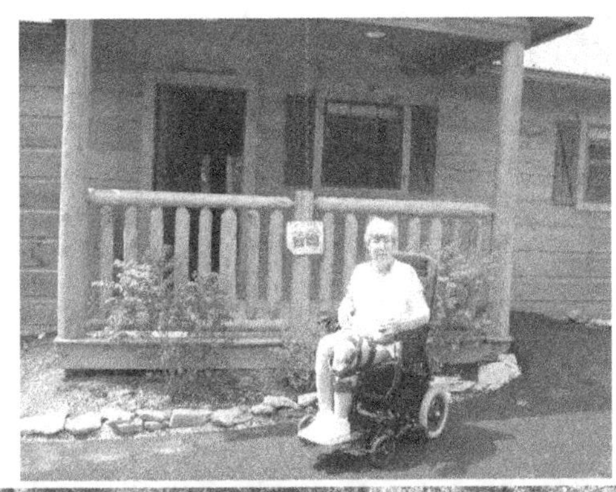

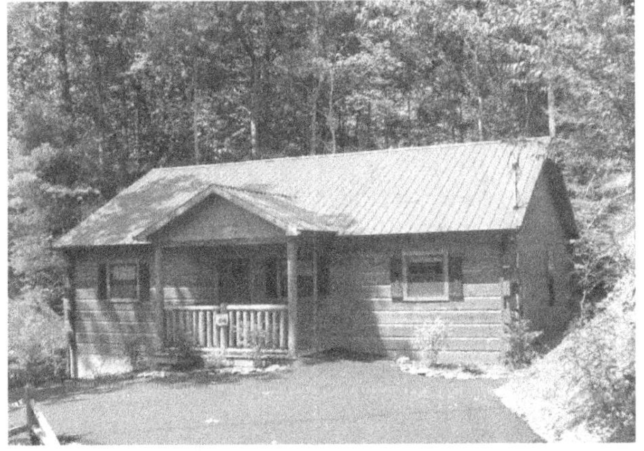

2006 to 2016

* * *

1. What adjustments have you made to accommodate your disability?
2. What plans do you need to think about for the future?
3. How do you handle these needs financially?

Paraphrase of Psalm 23 *by Phyllis*

1. The Lord is my Guide.
I shall not feel overwhelmed.

2. He helps me say, "no" at times; He lets
me catch my breath.

3. He's always with me; Continually do I
talk with Him.

4. When I feel overwhelmed and am
about to slip into depression, He is there
reassuring me.

5. His Word comforts me; He sends
friends to encourage me; I learn to trust
Him more and more.

6. Surely His presence will never leave
me, and I can depend on Him for the rest
of my life.

June 1996

* * *

1. Please consider writing your own paraphrase.
2. Is there someone you know who could profit from your
understanding and love, and who might need it today?
3. Write a list of things you're thankful for.

About the Author

From a farm in Michigan, to life in Florida, and then Tennessee. Phyllis grew up on a dairy farm north of Grand Rapids, Michigan and learned a strong work ethic there. She had polio at the age of 18 months and became a survivor and developed into a Type A personality. Both qualities continue to shape her life. Her faith is also a strong factor in her life.

She received a B.A. in speech at Central Michigan University; a M.A. in Instruction and Curriculum at Michigan State University; has taken post-graduate hours in English at Florida Atlantic University.

Her life has been lived as an educator: speech, forensics, drama, journalism, literature, and writing. She directed plays, coached debate and forensics, sponsored school newspapers. Her last position was as a writing adjunct at Nova University in Miami.

Because of Post-Polio syndrome, she had to quit teaching, but since that time she has published ten books (See Amazon.com) and gives writing workshops, encouraging others to share their stories—to leave a legacy for friends and family.

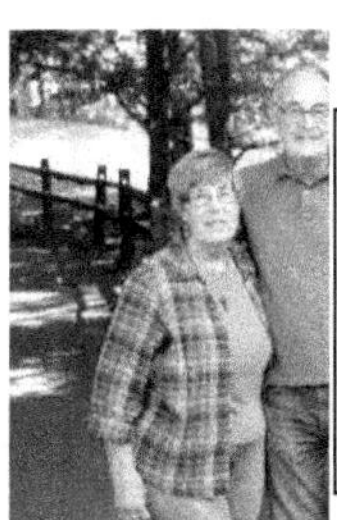

Phyllis with husband Ron

They celebrated their 50th wedding anniversary in 2016